I0075992

The Patient's Guide
Tumor Ablation

Adam E. M. Eltorai, MD, PhD
Matthew Czar Taon, MD, RPVI, WCC
Terrance T. Healey, MD

Praeclarus Press, LLC
©2020 Matthew Czar Taon. All rights reserved.

www.PraeclarusPress.com

Praeclarus Press, LLC
2504 Sweetgum Lane
Amarillo, Texas 79124 USA
806-367-9950
www.PraeclarusPress.com

DISCLAIMER
The information contained in this publication is advisory only and
is not intended to replace sound clinical judgment or individualized
patient care. The author disclaims all warranties, whether expressed
or implied, including any warranty as the quality, accuracy, safety,
or suitability of this information for any particular purpose.

ISBN: 978-1-946665-28-7
©2020 Matthew Czar Taon. All rights reserved.
Email: matthew.taon@gmail.com

Cover Design: Ken Tackett
Developmental Editing: Kathleen Kendall-Tackett
Copy Editing: Chris Tackett
Layout & Design: Nelly Murariu

CONTENTS

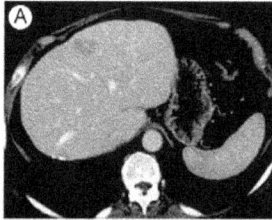

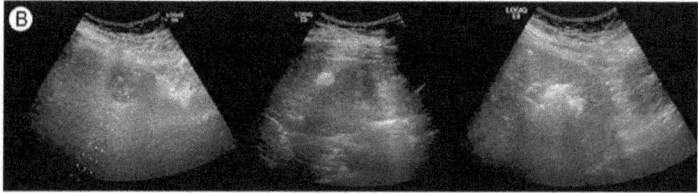

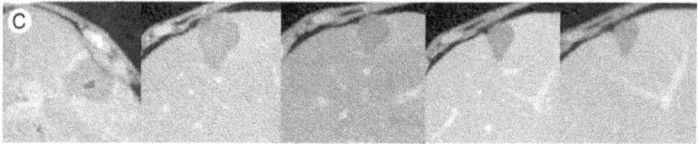

Microwave ablation for metastatic disease. Two gas-cooled microwave antennas were used. (A) Preablation CT. (B) Ultrasound images during procedure: before, early, and final. (C) Postablation CT images: day 0, 1 month, 6 months, and 12 months. CT, computed tomography.

WHAT IS "TUMOR ABLATION"?

Tumor ablation is a minimally-invasive method of destroying tumors without surgically removing them. Individual tumors can be destroyed using various forms of ablation, including heat (radiofrequency ablation, microwave ablation, high intensity focused ultrasound ablation), cold (cryoablation), electrical energy (irreversible electroporation), or chemical agents (percutaneous ethanol instillation).

For the most part, tumor ablation procedures are performed **percutaneously**, meaning "through the skin." Interventional physicians use imaging technology such as **ultrasound**, **live X-ray (fluoroscopy)**, **computer tomography (CT)**, or **magnetic resonance imaging (MRI)** to guide ablation devices directly to the site of a tumor. Many of these tumor ablation procedures use thin needles, approximately 1-2 mm in diameter, to get inside of or adjacent to a tumor to deliver their focused tumor destruction treatment. Alternatively, high intensity focused ultrasound (HIFU) ablation uses focused ultrasound energy to heat tumors to the point of destruction without the use of needles.

In essence, tumor ablation is a focused, minimally invasive, image-guided treatment that empowers interventional physicians to achieve optimal tumor destruction while minimizing injury to adjacent healthy tissue.

Why is a tumor ablation performed?

The goal of tumor ablation is to optimize tumor destruction while minimizing injury to healthy tissue. Ablative techniques can be used to destroy either benign (non-cancerous) or malignant (cancerous) tumors, depending on the patient's clinical scenario. Ablative therapies can be used to destroy tumors in many parts of the body, including, but not limited to, the liver, kidney, lung, and bones.

Often, the most definitive treatment of tumors is open surgical removal of the involved portions of the organ or the entire involved organ. However, many patients may not be candidates for open surgical treatment due to the extent or location of the disease or because their overall health would portend unacceptably high surgical risk. Ablative therapies are often used as an alternative to surgical resection for patients with few tumors. For patients with an increased number of tumors, or tumors involving multiple organs, systemic, whole-body treatment options such as chemotherapy may be more effective.

Tumor ablation can be performed with the intent of curing a patient's disease. However, even in cases where a complete cure may not be possible, ablative treatments can be used to improve the patient's quality of life by reducing the tumor burden.

The decision of whether an ablative treatment is appropriate for a patient's clinical scenario is best made after close communication between the patient and the patient's **multidisciplinary** medical team, which includes a medical oncologist, surgical oncologist, and interventional radiologist.

HOW DO I PREPARE FOR MY TUMOR ABLATION?

When discussing the possibility of tumor ablation with your interventional physician, it is important to report all medications or herbal supplements you may be taking. Depending on the clinical scenario, your physician may recommend that you stop taking some medications, such as blood-thinning medications, nonsteroidal anti-inflammatory medications (NSAIDS), or Metformin for a period of time prior to the procedure.

It is important to communicate any allergies or medication reactions you may have had in the past, including contrast allergies.

Women should communicate if there is any possibility that they may be pregnant. This is particularly important, since ablative procedures that use live X-ray (fluoroscopy) or CT may expose the fetus to radiation.

You may be recommended to visit a laboratory to obtain blood tests prior to a tumor ablation procedure. This is often done to assess kidney function and/or bleeding risk.

Depending on the time of your scheduled procedure, you may be instructed to avoid eating or drinking anything after midnight on the night prior to your procedure or after breakfast the day of your procedure

Your physician will instruct you as to which medications you may continue to take on the morning of your procedure. It is best to plan for a relative or friend to drive you home after your procedure. Once you arrive for your procedure, you will be asked to change into a gown. Removal of jewelry is recommended prior to the procedure.

WHAT IS THE EQUIPMENT LIKE?

Imaging equipment used to guide tumor ablation procedures includes ultrasound, live X-ray (fluoroscopy), computer tomography (CT), or magnetic resonance imaging (MRI).

An ultrasound machine is composed of a handheld probe that is connected to a specialized computer, and the picture is displayed on a high definition monitor. A fluoroscopy imaging unit is composed of a patient table, a movable X-ray device, and a high definition monitor to view the imaging in real-time.

A CT scanner is composed of a ring-like scanner and sliding exam table. The ring-like structure of the CT scanner contains devices that project and detect X-rays. The CT scanner uses a motorized, sliding table to move patients in and out of the machine. Often, this sliding table has a thick pad overlying it to provide patient comfort. A variety of pillows or foam tools may be used to optimize your positioning for the scan. Multiple scans will be performed throughout the procedure.

An MRI machine may be an open-ring or closed-ring configuration and also use a motorized, sliding table to move patients in and out of the machine. As with CT, multiple MRI scans will be performed throughout an ablation procedure.

There are various types of ablative treatments available. The decision as to what type of ablation device would be most effective depends on the patient's clinical history, anatomy, and disease manifestation.

Radiofrequency (RF) ablation uses thin, needle-like ablation electrodes to transmit an electric current from a radiofrequency generator directly into a tumor. This electric current creates focal areas of high temperature, which induce tumor cell death. Tumor cell death is often achieved at temperatures >45°C (113°F), with complete tumor necrosis occurring at >60°C (140°F).

Microwave (MW) ablation utilizes needle-like antennae to transmit microwaves directly into a tumor to create focal areas of high temperature that kill tumor cells.

High intensity focused ultrasound (HIFU) ablation utilizes MRI-imaging to guide a focused ultrasound beam to generate a lethal focus of heat at a single point within the body. This process is repeated as many times as is necessary until the target tissue is destroyed. Of note, HIFU uses an ultrasound transducer, similar to those used for diagnostic imaging, but with much higher energy to induce tumor cell death.

Cryoablation uses needle cryoprobes to produce extremely low temperatures in a tumor-containing area. Tumor cell death usually occurs at a temperature of less than -40 °C.

Irreversible electroporation uses needle-like electrodes to apply a high-voltage, low-energy direct current to a tumor. This causes the formation of pores in the tumor cell membranes, which induces tumor cell death.

Percutaneous ethanol instillation involves injecting absolute alcohol directly into a tumor via a thin needle. Alcohol destroys the membranes of tumor cells leading to tumor cell death.

WHAT DOES THE PROCEDURE INVOLVE?

Tumor ablations require careful positioning of devices to destroy tumor cells. Thus, it is important that patients are comfortable and completely still for the entirety of the procedure. Patients usually receive general anesthesia to ensure that they are completely still throughout the procedure. General anesthesia renders a patient completely unconscious and unable to feel pain during medical procedures. In some cases, general anesthesia may not be required, and local anesthesia with moderate/ conscious sedation may suffice. Moderate/conscious sedation is a type of sedation in which the patient is awake and able to tolerate procedures while maintaining his or her own cardiorespiratory function.

After the procedure, a bandage is placed over the tiny incision, and patients generally stay at the hospital overnight and can return home the next day.

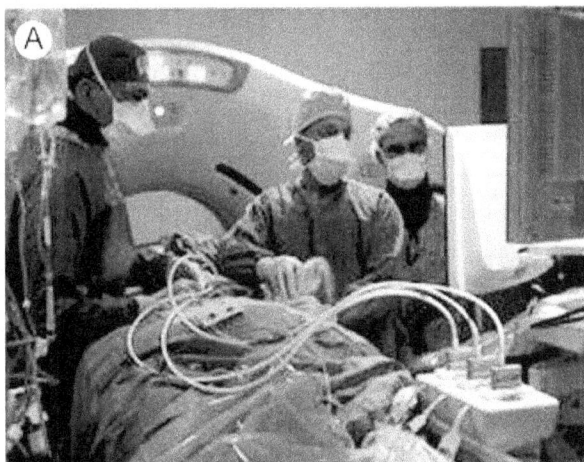

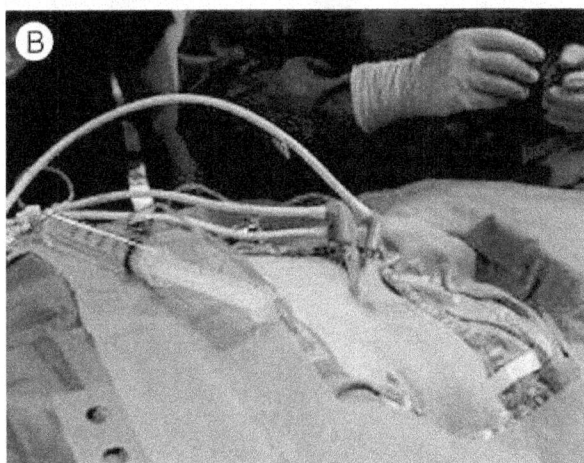

Images from within the ablation suite.
(A) Operator working together with ultrasound technologist.
(B) Insertion of 3 gas-cooled microwave antennas.
Hydrodissection was performed before ablation.
(Color version of figure is available online.)

Taken from https://www.ncbi.nlm.nih.gov/pmc/articles/PMC4281168/

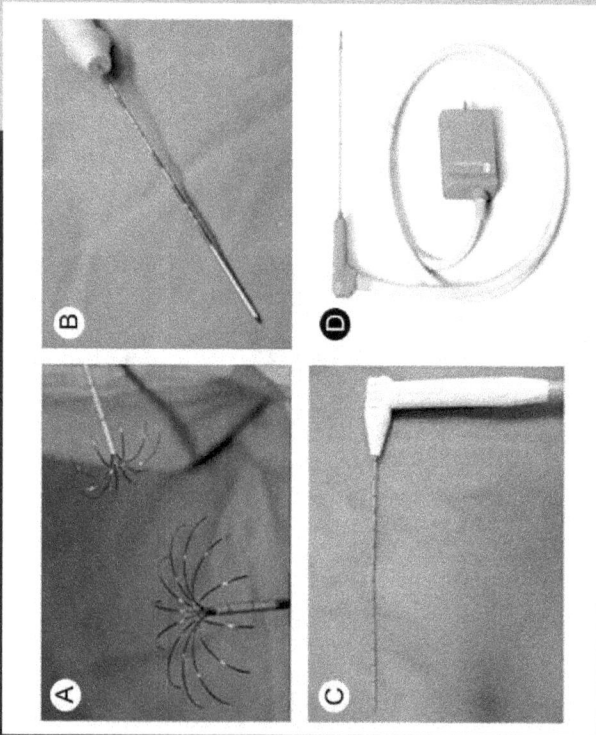

Thermal ablation applicators. (A) Deployable RF electrode, (B) single water-cooled RF electrode, (C) cryoprobe, and (D) gas-cooled microwave antenna. (Color version of figure is available online.)

WHAT DOES A TUMOR ABLATION FEEL LIKE?

The ablation procedure begins with the patient laying down on an examination table. Multiple monitoring devices will be attached to the body to assess vitals (blood pressure, heart rate, oxygenation) throughout the procedure.

The interventional physician will use imaging technology such as ultrasound, CT, or MRI to visualize the targeted tumor.

General anesthesia is utilized for most ablation procedures. Thus, patients are completely unconscious and unable to feel pain throughout the entirety of the procedure. Patients may feel pain or soreness at the tiny incision site where the ablation needles were placed. Also, patients may feel soreness in their throat due to the use of a breathing tube during general anesthesia.

What happens after the procedure?

Immediately after the procedure, patients are transferred from the procedure room to the recovery room. Pain or nausea related to the procedure can be controlled through intravenous (IV) or oral medications.

Many tumor ablation procedures can be performed in an outpatient setting where the patient is able to return home the same day or within 23 hours. Patients are usually able to return to their normal level of activity within a few days.

How will I know the results of my procedure?

Immediately after the procedure, you or your family will be updated with the results and further recommendations. Most interventional physicians will also schedule an outpatient clinic follow-up to discuss the next steps in the therapeutic plan.

WHAT ARE THE RISKS OF A TUMOR ABLATION? WHAT ARE THE BENEFITS?

Risks of any tumor ablation procedure include injury to adjacent healthy tissue. These can range in severity from unnoticeable injury to the extremely rare occurrence of patient death. Injury can occur due to the placement of the needle or as a result of the ablation itself. For example, if the needle traverses through the borders of the lungs, it can create a pneumothorax, an abnormal collection of gas in the chest cavity that collapses part of the lungs. If a blood vessel is injured, blood can leak into various cavities of the body.

If ionizing radiation, such as X-rays, is used for image guidance during the tumor ablation procedure, there are extremely rare risks of radiation injury or latent malignancy. As with any procedure where the skin is penetrated, there is a risk of infection requiring antibiotics. Lastly, there is a risk of incomplete or unsuccessful tumor destruction.

The primary benefit of tumor ablation is tumor destruction in a less invasive fashion. Interventional percutaneous tumor ablation generally takes less time to perform compared to open surgery. Lastly, ablation procedures tend to have reduced overall cost compared to other treatments.

ARE THERE LIMITATIONS TO A TUMOR ABLATION?

The primary limitation of tumor ablation is its dependence on adequate access to a tumor. For example, if a tumor is surrounded by critical organs, it would be difficult to access the tumor with an ablation needle probe. Furthermore, for tumors that are located deep within the patient's body, a needle probe may not be long enough to adequately access a patient's tumor.

FREQUENTLY ASKED QUESTIONS

Q: Does a tumor ablation involve any radiation?

A: It depends on what type of ablation is performed and what kind of imaging modality is used to guide the needle ablation. If X-rays are involved, there is ionizing radiation present.

Q: Are there any risks to a tumor ablation?

A: Yes, these are described above.

Q: How long will my tumor ablation procedure take?

A: It varies based on the study but usually less than an hour.

Q: When will I be able to go home?

A: Usually within the same day or within 23 hours.

GLOSSARY

ABLATION

Removal or destruction of a lesion.

PERCUTANEOUS

"Through the skin."

ULTRASOUND

Imaging modality that uses sound waves to visualize tissues within the body.

CT

An imaging modality that utilizes a ring-like scanning machine, a sliding exam table, and X-rays to produce high-quality images of the human body.

MRI

Magnetic resonance imaging utilizes a magnetic field to ascertain differences in the magnetic properties of human tissue and provide high-quality imaging of the human body.

MULTIDISCIPLINARY

Involving several medical specialties in an approach to a topic or problem.

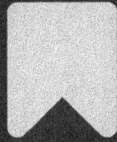

ADDITIONAL RESOURCES

Ablation for liver cancer-American
Cancer Society

https://www.cancer.org/cancer/liver-cancer/
treating/tumor-ablation.html

Extensive academic appraisal of the data
related to tumor ablation in different types of
tumors: Gandhi, Ripal T., Ganguli, Suvranu.
Practical guides in Interventional Radiology:
Interventional oncology. Thieme, 2016.

MY CONTACTS

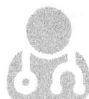

NAME

CONTACT

NAME

CONTACT

NAME

CONTACT

NAME

CONTACT

MY APPOINTMENTS

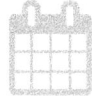

MONDAY

Date:
_____

TUESDAY

Date:
_____

WEDNESDAY

Date:
_____

THURSDAY

Date:
_____

FRIDAY

Date:
_____

SATURDAY

Date:
_____

MY QUESTIONS

MY QUESTIONS

MY QUESTIONS

MY QUESTIONS

MY QUESTIONS

MY NOTES

MY NOTES

MY NOTES

MY NOTES

MY NOTES

MY NOTES